Prepper's SHTF Stockpile

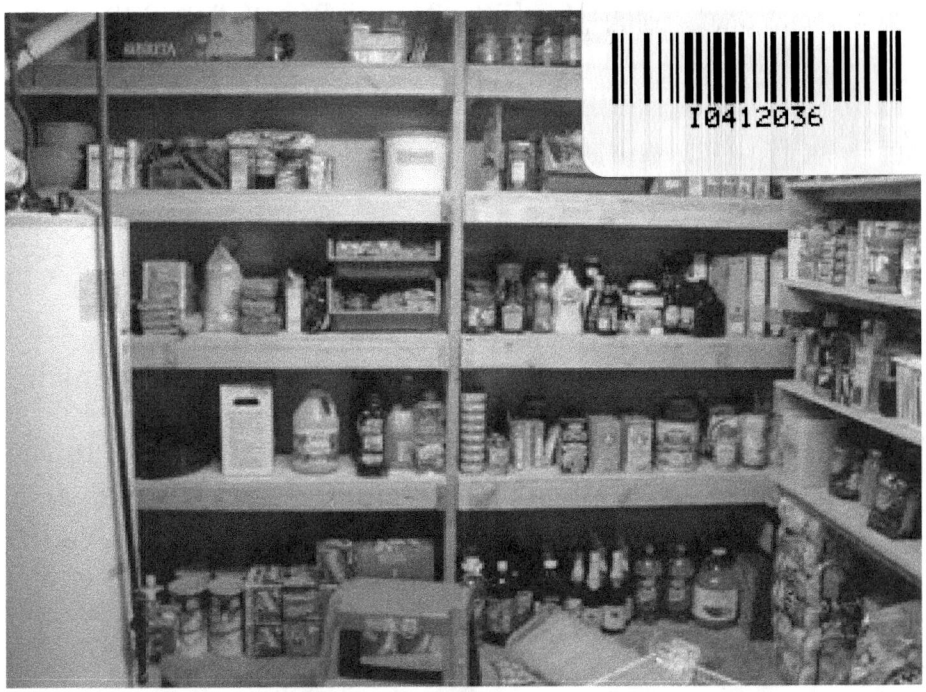

The Ultimate Disaster Preparedness And Survival Essentials Guide

By *Ron Johnson*

Disclaimer
This book is intended to be a general guide to raise awareness and to help people make informed decisions in the context of their own personal circumstance.
The author accepts no responsibility for any loss or injury, be it personal or financial, as a result for the use or misuse of the information in this book. If you have any doubts or concerns after reading this book, please speak to a qualified person before taking any actions.

Contents

Introduction

Chapter 1

The Basics Of Disaster Survival

Chapter 2

Ensuring You Have Enough Food

Chapter 3

Ensuring You Have Enough Water

Chapter 4

Shelter And Other Important Essentials

Chapter 5

Assembling The Ultimate First Aid Kit

Chapter 6

Dealing With Pets In A Disaster Situation

Conclusion

Introduction

You have seen it on television and done a little searching on the internet, but you still have a lot of questions about stockpiling for an emergency. That is only natural. Depending on what you read or what you saw, you may be a little confused and even a little wary. The idea of stockpiling has long been associated with those who were of a different mindset than the norm in society and you are worried about jumping on board something that could set you apart from your neighbours, family and friends.

You are different and that is perfect. You don't want to be like the rest of the people who assume nothing bad will ever happen and just go on with life with no thought for the future. You want to be the one who is paying attention to the world and what is happening. You want to be the one who is taking the time to put together a cache of goods and supplies that will keep you alive and well in the aftermath of catastrophe. Nobody ever knows when disaster will strike. Just because you live in an up scale neighbourhood and disaster has never stricken before, it doesn't mean it will never happen.

You need to get prepared. By creating a healthy stockpile of food, water, first aid and various other supplies, you are giving yourself the best shot at living after a natural disaster has rolled through or an act of war has crippled the nation. Those who chose not to prepare and didn't put together a stockpile of necessities will suffer and possibly perish. Those folks will be forced to wait and hope that help will arrive soon. They will have a much tougher time of it. If you didn't have to go through all of that, why would you?

This book is going to help you put together a stockpile of goods that will sustain you and your family for weeks, months or possibly even a year or more. If you have checked out other books about preparing to live through a disaster, you have probably noticed there is a heavy emphasis on stocking up on food. While that is certainly important, there are plenty of other aspects that must be included in your survival preparation. This book covers it all. You will learn some of the most basic tricks to surviving if you have to abandon your home and head out into the wilderness.

This is the book that covers all areas of surviving a disaster and doesn't focus on any single aspect. This is the guide that could just save your life.

Chapter 1
The Basics Of Disaster Survival

No one can forget the catastrophe that struck the Philippines on the 8th day of November in 2013. Super Typhoon Haiyan brought with it strong and powerful winds, massive downpour of heavy rain, and a deadly storm surge which instantly took away thousands of innocent lives,

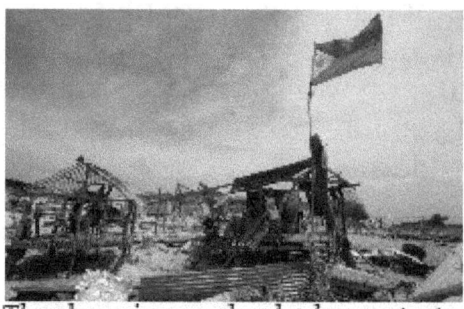

The above image clearly demonstrates the level of devastation caused by Typhoon Haiyan in 2013 which claimed about 2600 lives

destroyed millions of crops and animals, ravished thousands of acres of properties, and left the Philippines helpless and horror struck. With a record of 6 landfalls, it was the greatest and deadliest typhoon to be ever recorded in all of history.

However, there were experts who said that the great number of fatalities during the Typhoon Haiyan was not caused by the typhoon itself, but the lack of proper preparation. If the people were properly warned about the storm surge and if they were trained beforehand to prepare for the upcoming calamity, the number of dead people could have been lessened.

This just goes to show that preparing for a calamity can be the difference between life and death.

This chapter will talk about the basics of disaster survival and what to do and prepare before, during, and after a calamity or disaster.

THE BASICS

If there is going to be an upcoming natural calamity like a storm or a hurricane, the government will usually inform the public as early as possible through news and other means of public declarations. However, typhoons and storms like Haiyan are just a few of the natural disasters that people can be hit with and can paralyse our normal daily routines. Aside from storms, there are also earthquakes, volcanic eruptions, forest fires, tornadoes, hurricanes, hail storms, tsunamis, flash floods, and storm surges –all of which can put us in grave danger, destroy our prized possessions, and take our loved ones away from us.

Not only natural disasters can put us in great danger but disasters caused by man can leave us vulnerable too. Wars, fires, robberies, and cases of kidnapping can also pose great threats to our lives.

So, it is imperative that we know the what, when, where, and how of survival. These are the four basic questions that can save you and your family from the deadly effects of disasters.

The What

What to prepare

Here is a list of the items that you should put in your survival kit and the items that you must purchase beforehand in case of emergencies.

- Water supply that is adequate for the entire family and can last up to a minimum of 7 days.

- A supply of non-perishable foods that is adequate for the entire family and can last up to a minimum of 7 days.

- A first-aid kit complete with the medications taken by the members of the family and other medical supplies such as asthma inhalers, a nebulizer, and a thermometer.

- Battery-operated transistor radios with extra batteries. Solar powered radios can be included to save batteries.

- At least one flashlight for each member of the family with extra batteries. LED or solar powered flashlights are also encouraged since these are durable and offer powerful illumination.

- Toiletries for the whole family such as soap, shampoo, toothbrushes, and toothpastes.

- A map of your city or province or country which will aid you in navigation in the case of evacuation.

- Extra blankets and towels for each member of the family.

- Whistles which can provide alternative sources of communication. A single blow of a whistle can serve as a signal or a guide to find a member of the group. It can also alert others to one's location.

- Matches or lighters are very important and should be present in every survival kit. They enable you to start a fire if need be. If you opt for matches, make sure that you keep them in zip-lock bags to prevent them from getting wet.

- Rain coats, umbrellas, and boots for every member of the family. These not only protect everyone from the rain, but also the cold.

- Spare clothing, jackets, underwear, hats, socks, and rubber shoes for every member of the family.

- Sleeping bags, tents, or hammocks that can accommodate the entire family.
- Scissors, knives, can openers, and other tools. A Swiss knife is a better investment since it contains a lot of tools and is very portable. These can all serve as tools and weapons for self-protection against predators.

- Utensils.

- Cash.

- Mobile phones, a netbook, or a laptop with chargers or power banks.

- A copy of your personal documents such as your license, passports, identification cards, and credit cards Keep all of these in a safe and dry place. These are all needed in case you have to exit the country or abandon your area quickly.

- Car keys and house keys.

- Small foldable chairs.
- Walkie-talkies will be your substitutes when your

mobile phone batteries run out and there's no electricity.

- If you have pets or babies, pack up necessary essentials for them as well, like collars, leashes, canned food, and bowls for pets and milk bottles, baby formula, vitamins, and plenty of diapers for babies. Pets and babies require extra care so make sure that you are ready for their every need.

- A compass, which is very helpful in times of survival, especially when you are lost.

- Bicycles with padlocks, preferably foldable ones because they are more portable and easy to keep. It is difficult to cruise the streets using your car during calamities such as storms and floods. Having bikes can allow you and your family to get moving without getting caught up in traffic or having to stop once in a while for gas. Bikes offer your family easy transport especially when you have to leave your area quickly.

- Inflatable floating devices which can help during floods and storms.

- Water proof bags and containers to ensure that your clothes, documents, and supplies are dry and protected from rain or extreme heat.

Always keep in mind that you can only touch these supplies during emergencies and when you actually use them, do not forget to replenish your supplies after for future needs. It would also be best if you group similar items together like tools and utensils and keep them in specific containers with labels. Put your survival kit in an accessible place to ensure easy retrieval during times of trouble.

What to do

- ## *Before*

    Your chance of surviving a disaster will increase if you really prepare for it in advance. Listed are some of the things that you need to do before a calamity.

    > **Keep watch.** Monitor the news for public announcements and instructions about where get food or water and where to go in the case of evacuation. Always stay alert and watch out for essential information that can help you identify the things that you still need to prepare. If you're faced with a hurricane, constantly check for information about the hurricane like how fast it is, how strong it is, where it is going, and what are the major areas that will be badly hit. If you're hit by an earthquake, know its intensity and magnitude as well as its centre.

    > **Check your supplies.** Check and monitor the expiration dates of your food and water supply regularly. Also, check for their qualities from time to time.

    > **Ready your supplies.** If it is already certain that your area will be hit by a hurricane or a storm, ready your supplies in advance and keep them within arm's reach so that you will not have trouble finding them. This can save you time, effort, and energy.

- > **Do some drills.** Always keep this mind-set: Practice makes perfect. It would be a lot easier if the members of your family already know what to do in times of trouble and master the procedure for survival, which can only be achieved through constant practice. You can save time and effort or even cheat death if all of your loved ones will stand by the drill and follow it. It would also be helpful if you educate your children about map and compass reading for easy navigation or teach the older members of the family how to operate certain gadgets and tools. Teach everyone how to make fire from leaves and the rays of the sun. Train everyone how to do basic first aid, knot tying, and shelter building. These set of skills will really come in handy in time of emergencies.

- > **Make a plan.** Draw maps and itineraries for the family in case the members will have to be separated from each other. Agree upon meeting places and hide-outs that only the family know of to ensure everybody's safety and that everyone will really find each other. Plan out short cuts and routes to get to the meeting places faster and easier.

- *During*
- > **Keep calm.** Panic is the leading cause of death because when you panic, you cannot think properly. Even if you are nervous, try to inhale, exhale, relax, and remember the things that you should do. If there is a storm, stay indoors and don't come out until it's already safe to do so. If there is an earthquake, seek protection under sturdy tables or chairs. If you can't

exit the building, go under the door frame because it is the strongest structure that is guaranteed to be left standing in case the building crumbles down. When in an open space or field, cover your head to prevent getting hit by falling debris. In case of fires, crawl down towards the exit to prevent suffocation. You will not be able to do this if you panic and decide to run around the place with no direction to go to.

- **Stay connected.** Constant communication is the key to ensuring everyone's safety. Try as much as possible to reach your loved ones and know their whereabouts in case you get separated from them.

- **Check for damages.** Check your roofs, windows, doors, gates, and electric lines for possible causes of fire or harm.

- **Stay tuned to the news.** Get information and updates about the calamity that you are facing.

- *After*
- **Do a count off.** Be sure to have all of the members accounted for. Make sure everyone is safe and with the group. If someone is missing, search for him or her quickly.
- **Assess your supplies.** Make sure that you still have enough to keep you going for a few more days until everything goes back to normal. Replenish exhausted supplies and fix or replace broken gadgets and tools.

- **Help others.** There may be other people who might need your help. Make the effort to help out those who got hit by a calamity badly and participate in relief operations.

The When

When should I prepare?
- **As early as possible.** It would even be best if you prepare ahead of time even if there's no calamity yet. Always remember that prevention is better than cure.

When should I replace my supplies?
- **Regularly.** You must know the expiration dates of your canned goods, your batteries, bottled supplies, and other goods in order to avoid using spoiled supplies at times of calamities. You must also replace broken tools and gadgets as soon as possible in order to ensure that they will work when you need them to.

The Where

Where should I go?
- **Stay at home.** Do not go out until it's already safe. However, if your home is not a safe place to stay and you need to seek shelter some place else, go to the nearest evacuation centre that the government has provided. During storms, avoid going to the beach or places near bodies of water. During earthquakes, go to open spaces and protect your head. During fires, run away from the source and keep yourself oxygenated. During tsunamis or storm surges, go to high places like mountains or hills and stay away

from seas or oceans.

Where will I ask for help?

- **Hospitals and organizations.** Go to the hospital as fast as you can if you or any member of the family is badly hurt. You can also ask for help from agencies such as the Red Cross. Also, be updated of the locations of groups who will hand out relief goods and free check-ups.

Where should I keep my survival kit?

- **Only you and your family knows.** Keep your kits in accessible places or secret locations that only the members of the family know.

The how's of survival like how to make fire, how to find food and water, and how to make an improvised shelter will be tackled in the succeeding chapters.

Chapter 2

Ensuring You Have Enough Food

We all need food in order to survive. We get the necessary nutrients and minerals that our bodies need from the food that we consume every single day. Thankfully, we get to eat each day since food is readily available in our environment. We can get fruits and vegetables in our gardens or in supermarkets. When we are hungry, we can easily go to a restaurant or to a fast food chain and order what we want to eat. However, during the times of calamity or when a disaster strikes, food is one of the things that might become unavailable to us. There is a possibility that our supply of food would be cut off and inaccessible. How, then, can we gain access to food when going to a restaurant or purchasing food from the supermarket is not possible?

This chapter is dedicated to food supply and it will teach you how to have your own food when you are caught up in a calamity.

What kinds of food to keep

Here are the qualities that you should consider when preparing your own food supply:

• Your food must have a long shelf life.

When a disaster strikes your area, it will be expected that cooking food or even buying it from the grocery will be a great challenge and, at times, may even be impossible. That is why it is better to store foods that don't easily spoil or rot and is very easy to prepare like canned goods, instant noodles, or energy bars. These kinds of food can alleviate hunger and can give you energy but only requires little or minimal cooking. These will also last for days or even weeks. The advantage of keeping non-perishable food is that it can keep your family going for days and you can easily prepare them even if you are in a disadvantageous location or circumstance (for

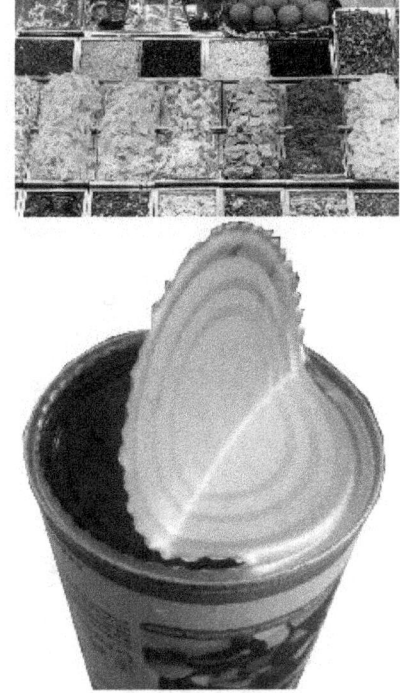

Canned and dried food are great food sources as they are portable, require no electricity to keep fresh, will last a long time and usually require little preparation to consume

example, you have no electricity or you evacuated to the mountain). They also last for a long time which makes it possible to store them without the aid of a refrigerator.

• Food which does not provoke an allergic reaction.

Your food supply would be of not much help if most of your family members can't eat it due to health issues and allergies. Take into consideration your family's health background when shopping for food supply. Make sure that the things you purchase are not bad for their health.

• **Neither salty nor spicy.**

Avoid having spicy or salty foods in your food supply for they can cause us to drink an excess of water. During a calamity, water can also be a scarce resource so you and your family must save and conserve it.

Where to keep your food supply

There are a couple of factors that you must consider when storing and stashing your food away in order to make sure that the your food will not be easily spoiled and the shelf life of your provisions will be lengthened.

• **Sunlight**

Do not place your food supply under direct sunlight. Extreme temperature can spoil food since light can cause deteriorative reactions to the constituents in food.

• **Humidity**

Humid atmospheres can also spoil and decrease the shelf life of canned goods since it can promote the growth of microorganisms that can cause spoilage.

• **Temperature**

You should store food in a cool and dry place. This is the ideal temperature that can help lengthen the shelf life of your food supply.

• **Presence of rodents and other pests**

Keep your supply away from pests such as rats and insects. These organisms may destroy your supply and even consume all of it.

Ideal storage places for food supply

The rule of thumb here is that you should keep your supply in a safe and accessible place where all the members of the family knows. Ideal places can include cabinets and cupboards. You can even keep it in drawers or in plastic containers to keep rodents away and to maintain the temperature of storage place.

How to properly store your food supply

.   Make sure that your supply will last for at least 1 week and will be adequate for the whole family.

.   Keep your canned goods and dried supply of food in a cool, dark, and dry place or in containers that are appropriately labelled.

.   Avoid getting your food in contact with petroleum products like gasoline to prevent contamination and poisoning.

.   Always monitor the expiry dates of canned goods and other dried food.

Items to prepare for cooking food

.   Portable pans, pots, and ladles.

.   Can openers, bottle openers, knives, spoons, and forks.

.   Plastic plates and cups.

.   A small portable stove with some extra cans of butane

as source of fuel.

Finding food supply in the wilderness

If ever you find yourself in the wilderness or if you have to evacuate to the mountains or the forest to avoid a disaster, it may be very difficult to find food and prepare food. If this ever happens, you can search the area for fruit trees or edible plants. Do not harvest any suspicious fruit and make sure that you don't eat poisonous berries or leaves or vines. Always double check before popping anything into your mouth.

If you don't have any cooking material or a portable stove with you, you can make an improvised stove using medium sized stones. Place the stones on top of one another until you can form a semi-circular wall and put your pot on top. Gather some dry firewood to fuel the fire.

Surviving in the wilderness is in our nature. Our ancestors used to be gatherers and hunters during the ancient times and they have successfully passed on the genes that aid survival in the wilderness. All we have to do is to rekindle our once forgotten knowledge about nature and harness it in order to help us survive during extreme emergencies.

Food must be one of the top priorities when preparing for a disaster since it is needed by all of us to ensure our survival--but it is not the only priority. Water is very important too. Water supply will be tackled in the next chapter.

Chapter 3

Ensuring You Have Enough Water

Although food is an important aspect of survival, water is more important. You can survive a few days without eating a meal but you will not live to see another day if you will not drink water for 24 hours straight. This is because our body is mostly composed of water and we lose a lot of this water when we sweat, urinate, spit, remove bowels, or cry. We have to replenish the amount of water that we lose every single day in order to prevent dehydration which can cause illness or even death.

During calamities and disasters, the water supply can be cut off to and water can become inaccessible due to a very high demand and a low supply. It is possible that the water supply in an area might not be enough for everyone especially during droughts and La Niña. It is also possible that the main source of the water supply in an area is contaminated especially during floods and storms.

This chapter is about gaining access to water supply and will teach you how to have your own supply of water during calamities.

Planning your own emergency water supply

- You must allocate 1 gallon of drinking water a day for every person or pet in the family. Allocate more for the members who have illnesses or for those who are taking medications.

- Make sure that your supply of drinkable water will

last for at least one week per person or pet.

- Six pails of water for hygiene must be allocated per day for at least one week.

- Also store either chlorine, bleach, or iodine to disinfect water.

How to make sure that your water supply is safe to drink

It is not only important to have a water source during calamities but it is also important that you are sure that your water source is safe to drink and use. Having access to clean water during calamities and disasters can be very difficult so here are some ways to follow so that you can make sure that you will not get amoebiasis or diarrhoea from drinking your stored water.

- **Buy bottled and purified bottles.** This is the safest option for you. Buying purified drinking bottles can be a little expensive but at least you are sure that you and your family are drinking clean and safe water. The

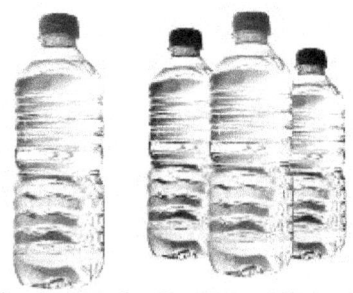

In the event of a short-term disaster bottled water is one of of the safest and most effective water sources, bottles water comes in various sized so be sure to keep a variety of sizes to suit the various disasters which may occur.

empty bottles can even be used as an improvised floating device which you can use during floods or storms.

- **Sanitize the containers of your water.**
  Sanitizing the containers of your drinking water is the first thing that you should do if you are fortunate enough to still have a supply of water during a calamity. Doing so can prevent bacteria and germs from contaminating your water supply. First, wash your containers with dish washing soap and rinse water. Next, mix a teaspoon of chlorine or bleach with one quart of water and wash the inner part of the containers using this solution. Shake the containers properly so that the solution can cover every area. Wait for 30 minutes before rinsing them with water. Lastly, let the containers dry before filling them with water.

- **Purify your water using iodine.** Purifying your water source is very simple. All you have to do is add 5 to 10 drops of iodine tincture solution, which is 2% iodine and 47% alcohol, into 32 ounces or 1 litre of water. Wait for 5 minutes before turning your container upside down in order to purify its upper area as well. Wait for another 30 minutes and then taste your water.

- **Boil.** You can heat or boil your water in order to kill off harmful bacteria and germs that can contaminate your water supply.

Storing your water supply properly

Just like food, you have to properly store your water as well to prevent contamination or poisoning. Here are some tips that you can follow in order to keep your drinking water safe to drink:

- **Label every container.** This will help you identify which containers store drinking water and water for cleaning. It will also avoid confusion on which containers hold gasoline or fuel and which containers hold clean water.

- **Keep your water in a place with a constant and cool temperature.** Avoid placing your water supply in an area where it can be hit by direct sunlight. Doing so can help maintain the coolness and freshness of your drinking water.

- **Avoid storing your water supply near toxic chemicals.** This is to avoid your water from getting contaminated and poisoned by harmful chemicals.

Alternative sources of drinking water

During extreme circumstances and situations, it is important that you know where to find alternative sources of drinking water to help you survive. You can use rain water, for example, to wash the dishes and your utensils. You can even use the rain to flush the toilet or clean your body. You can also locate bodies of water to get clean and pure drinking water. You must know where the nearest river or lake or stream is so you can get drinking water from these bodies of water in case you really don't have any access to drinkable water. If you are not satisfied with the cleanliness of the water coming from lakes and streams, you can always purify it using bleach, chlorine, or iodine. You must be careful when getting water from rivers especially during storms though. The current can be very rough and fast and it can take you along with it.

Now, you already know how to prepare and get access to the supply of food and water. But how about shelter? How can we protect ourselves from calamities if ever we have to abandon our homes? The next chapter will answer these questions.

Chapter 4

Shelter And Other Important Essentials

A shelter is our main protection from harmful elements of the environments. It shields us from the burning rays of the sun, cold blow of the wind, destructive pour of the rain, and threats posed by predators, both humans and animals. However, our shelter can be destroyed during calamities too and there are times when our homes are not safe enough for us to stay in during disasters.

This chapter is about making improvised shelters and seeking safe places where you can seek refuge into during calamities and disasters. This will also discuss preparing the appropriate clothing during disasters, how to make fire, and what gadgets and weapons will help you survive during calamities.

Shelters

You must be ready to abandon your house when you need to. You must know how to make your own tent if you don't have any. You must know how to find a perfect and safe place to set your camp in. If you don't know how to do any of these, don't worry. Here are some of the things to consider when building your very own shelter:

- **Type of shelter that you need.** If you are making a shelter for one person only, you can try to make the simple "one man shelter". It can be made using only a tree, a pole and something that can serve as a canopy. All you have to do is incline or slant the pole against a tree's trunk and the ground. Secure both ends of the pole with some rope or some nails. Finally, hang a water proof blanket or anything that can serve as a canopy on the pole and fasten the ends of the canopy on the ground using some nails or rocks. If you are building a shelter for a family of four, you can tie a rope that connects two tree trunks and hang a large canopy on the rope. Fasten the ends of the canopy on the ground using rocks and nails. What's important is that the shelter that you will build must protect everyone from the rain and the heat of the sun.

- **The kind of materials available.** There are a lot of materials that you can utilize in order to make a shelter. All you have to do is make some improvisations and let your creativity work. You can make a roof out of large leaves, twigs, and branches. You can use cardboard boxes as a floor or a sleeping mat. You can use plastic chairs in order to make a simple fort. If you just let your brain do some magic, you will actually find things that you can use in order to make an improvised but sturdy shelter.

- **Time and effort.** If you have to make a shelter quickly and you have no one else to help you, don't try to make a sophisticated one. Just keep it simple but remember to make sure that your shelter is safe and clean.

Appropriate Clothing

During disasters, it would be hilarious to wear a bikini or a long gown paired with stilettos. You must dress accordingly in order to protect yourself from the sun and the rain and to help you move freely and comfortably.

In cases of typhoons and storms, you must wear jackets, raincoats, boots and thick clothing to prevent you from catching a cold or a fever. Wear clothes that are efficient in trapping heat to help you feel warm for prolonged hours.

When evacuating, make sure that you wear comfortable clothes that will not restrain your movements. Make sure that you can walk for miles, run, jump, or crawl in the clothes that you wear. Also have a satchel wherein you can keep tiny but essential knick knacks , a pair of sunglasses, caps, and shoes.

Making Fire

If you don't have a match or lighter with you, it will be a great challenge to make a fire. However, you must really learn how to do it manually. You can start a fire by gathering dried leaves and putting them under a bottle of water or a magnifying glass. Make sure that the rays of the sun will directly hit the bottle of the magnifying glass so that the heat can be refracted to the dried leaves. Continue doing this until the dried leaves start to smoke. You can also make fire by rubbing two surfaces of rocks together until you form a spark and ignite the dried leaves.

Gadgets And Weapons

Make sure that you have your mobile phones, walkie talkies, or compasses with you. It can also help if you have a water proof watch and a GPS system to help you tell time and know your location. Also keep a hand knife wherever you go in case when you have to cut something loose or you have to protect yourself from harmful animals or people with bad intentions.

Chapter 5

Assembling The Ultimate First Aid Kit

Image by Arria Belli

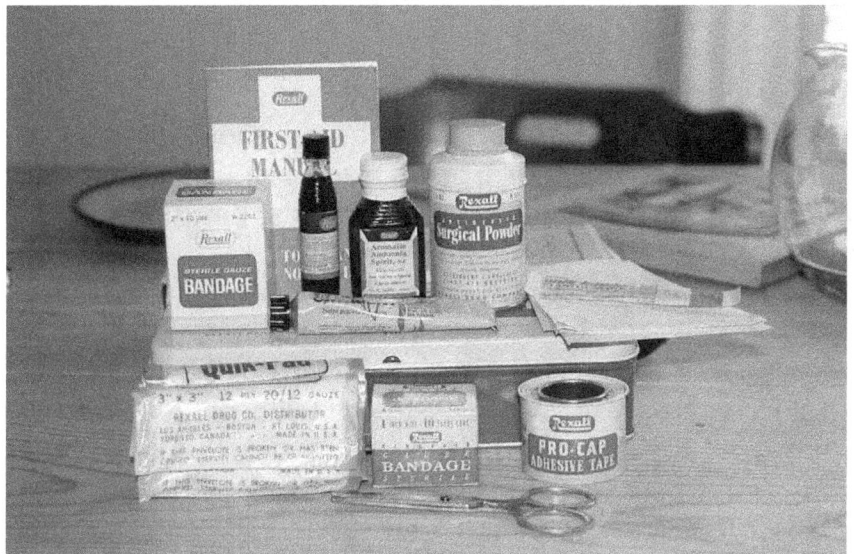

Above Image shows what the most basic self- assembled first aid kit should include

During disasters, you might be faced with certain emergencies that, if not remedied quickly, might progress into something serious and fatal. Also, you might have a difficulty in going immediately to the hospital and asking for help. With these possibilities, you must have a first-aid kit with you as a part of your survival kit in order to aid simple wounds, cuts, or illnesses.

This chapter will let you know the essential things that must be present in a prepper's first-aid kit.

Medications

You must have over-the-counter antibiotics, antivirals, analgesics, and anti-inflammatory drugs to aid bacterial and viral infections. You must also have treatments for cough, colds, flu, fever, LBM, hyperacidity, allergies, and stomach ache. Assess the health needs of your family and include their medications in your first aid kit.

Medical tools and supplies

You must also have basic medical tools such as clean and sterilized syringes, tourniquet, cotton balls, surgical scissors, gauze, medical tapes, bandages, band aids, alcohol, antiseptic solution, and clean gloves.

It is not enough to have these things in your kit. You must also learn how to do basic first-aid like CPR, Heimlich manoeuvre, treating sprains and twists, and bandaging and wound dressing. All of the items of your kit will be useless if you don't know how to use them properly and what first-aid treatments to apply on specific kinds of illnesses.

Chapter 6

Dealing With Pets In A Disaster Situation

As it has been said a while back, not only humans need saving during disaster and calamities. Our household pets are vulnerable to these threats too. In fact, they easily become stressed when there are calamities. That is why you must also prepare for the safety of your furry and cute friends.

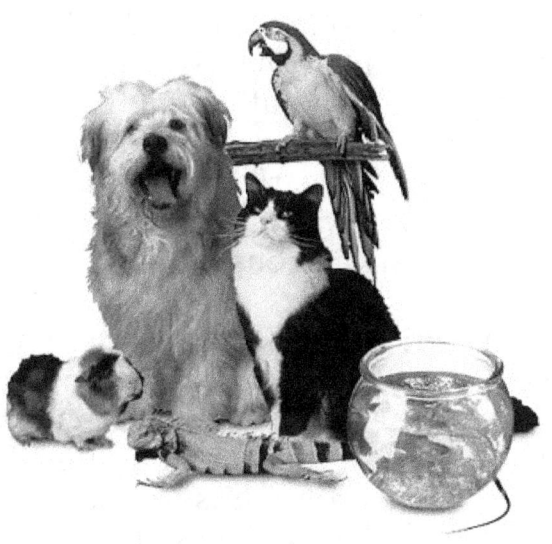

Make sure that your pets have their own water and food supply that can last up to a week. Make sure that you pack up some extra leashes and collars to avoid them from getting separated from you. Make sure that your pets have name tags and your address so that they can be quickly returned to you in case you lose them during your evacuation. Also provide a safe and clean shelter for them when you decide to evacuate. Like you, they can easily catch illnesses so make sure that you have medications for them too.

Basically, the things that you prepare for yourself and your family must also be the things that you prepare for your pets. Do not leave them helpless and vulnerable. If you take care of them properly, they might also return the favour and save you when you need help.

Conclusion

You have just taken in a lot of information and now you have a lot to think about. The key is not to get hung up on getting everything done today. This is a process that will take some time. That is why it is so important you start today and don't put it off until next week or next month when you have more time. Time is never guaranteed. Even if disaster does strike a month into your preparation process, you will still be better off than you would have been if you had done nothing.

Don't put off the planning. Building up supplies will take some time, but you can sit down today and start planning what you will do should disaster strike. Coming up with a plan will save you from the panic that so commonly takes hold when a storm hits or when things get a little scary in the world. You don't have to worry about what you will do— you already know. Your family already knows and you can spring into action rather than sit around or run in circles trying to figure out how to respond.

Take some time to make your plan and add a few supplies to your stockpile every week. Slowly building up your emergency stash will keep you from going into debt and from making quick, impulse purchases that won't do you a lot of good. Come up with a shopping list and make a commitment to add something new every week. Preparing for survival is the first step in living through whatever may come your way.

There is a lot to be done, but trying to do it all at once can frustrate you and you will likely give up and simply adopt the attitude you will take your chances. You don't have to do it all. Follow the instructions in this book and slowly build up your supply of food, water and supplies that will keep you alive. You will have peace of mind and be able to sleep better at night knowing you are ready for anything.

Good luck to you and happy prepping!

From The Author

Thank you for taking the time to read this book. As an author, I understand the importance of creating books which my readers will find both enjoyable and informative. If you have the time and feel generous, please don't hesitate to leave an honest review of this book.........Ron Johnson

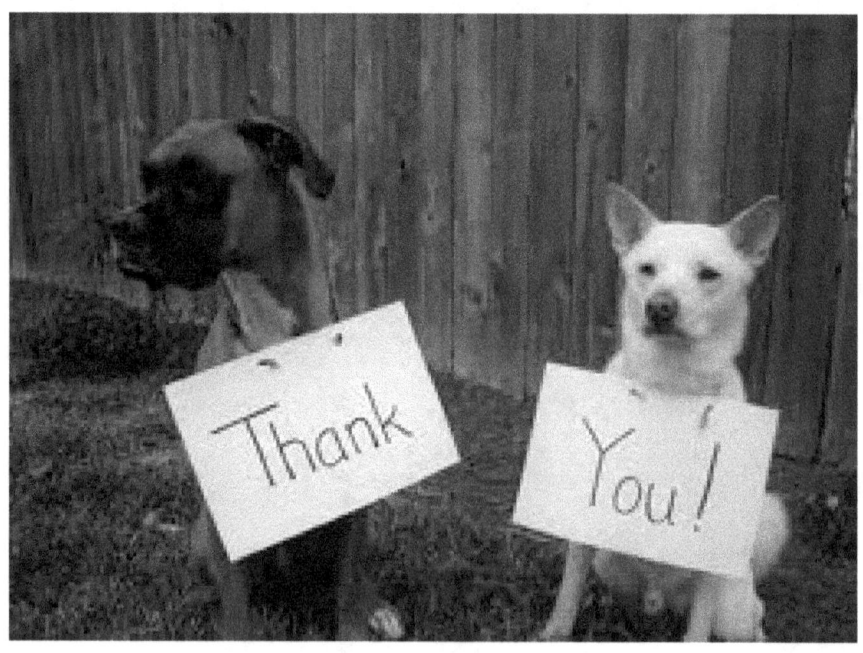

Other Books By Ron Johnson

<u>Prepper's Pantry</u>

In the event of an emergency having an adequate supply of food could mean the difference between life and death!

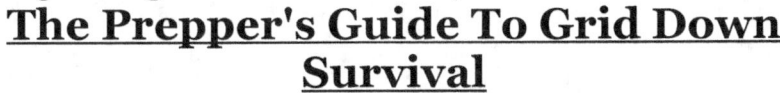

Are you prepared for any disaster that is about to happen? Do you already have emergency supplies? Is it enough to sustain you and your family's life for an extended period, when help from others would be close to impossible? Have you discussed and implemented the emergency plans with your family?

Fighting for your survival during times of disaster is not about luck, it's about the right knowledge that will help you pull through it. It is all about saving you and your family's life, with the tips provided in this book. Guess what? YOU CAN MAKE IT HAPPEN by reading and following all the guidelines laid out in my book.

<u>The Prepper's Guide To Grid Down Survival</u>

Are you ready to live through a long term downed power grid situation?

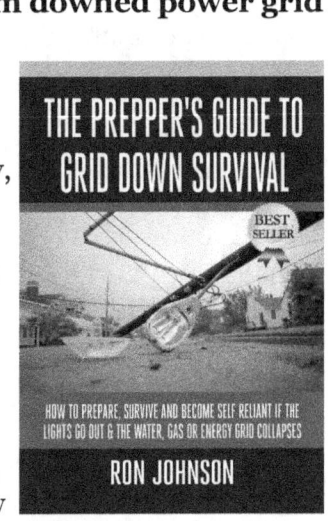

Many people don't stop to think how they will eat, get clean drinking water or stay warm when the power goes out. Unfortunately, the possibility of a widespread power failure that extends weeks or months is a very real possibility. This book covers some of the most plausible scenarios as well as how you will manage during the grid failure.

You need to think about how you will maintain personal hygiene, take care of toilet issues and feed your family as well as how you will keep them safe and warm. You don't know how much you rely on electricity until it is ripped away from you. It can leave your entire world turned upside down if you are not ready. It is hard to imagine and prepare for every little thing without doing some research first. This book will hold your hand and help you come up with a plan that will get you through a long lasting grid failure. Planning and preparing can help remove the fear that is associated with the unknown. Get your family involved and start your preparations with the help of the information in this book.

The Prepper's Guide To Off The Grid Survival

Have you dreamed of leaving your fast-paced, high stress world for one that is more laid back?

Do you want to leave behind the financial hardships of working day in and day out and barely making enough to put food on the table? If you answered yes, living off the grid is the answer! Getting off the grid and transitioning to a self-sustaining lifestyle that gives you financial freedom is one way for you to enjoy life more.

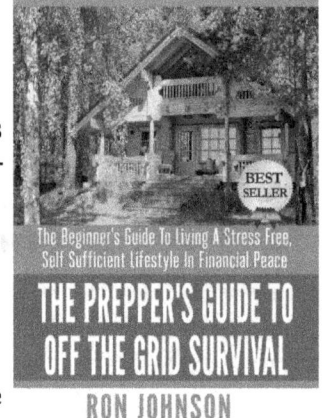

Learning how to grow your own food and living without some of the luxuries in life will give you financial peace of mind without destroying your quality of life. When you make the leap to going off the grid and relying only on the sun for your energy needs, you are making a conscious choice to do something good for the environment and your bank account. Raising livestock on your own land is one way to ensure your food is healthy as well as extremely cheap! The satisfaction of knowing you can provide for yourself without relying on city and government services is worth every penny of the initial investment to go off the grid. This book will help you make decisions about what you need to go off the grid and thrive.

www.ingramcontent.com/pod-product-compliance
Lightning Source LLC
Chambersburg PA
CBHW070517290526
45790CB00003B/1250